THE
OTHER
PMS

THE OTHER PMS

Your Survival Guide for
Perimenopause & Menopause

DR. LAKEISCHA W. MCMILLAN

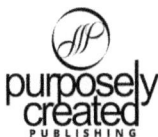

purposely
created
PUBLISHING

THE OTHER PMS
Published by Purposely Created Publishing Group™
Copyright © 2020 LaKeischa W. McMillan

All rights reserved.

Printed in the United States of America

ISBN: 978-1-64484-249-2

This book is dedicated to my husband, Wendell II, and our children, Wendell III and Skylar Nicole. Wendell, you have always been there to support me, and I love you. Wendell and Skylar, you all are my why, and Mommy loves you all so much.

This book is also dedicated to my family of origin: Mommy (Linda L. Webb), Daddy (the late Norton H. Webb, Sr.), and my little brother (Norton H. Webb, Jr.) —all 6'4" of you. You all have always been in my cheering section and I love you for it!

Table of Contents

Introduction

Growing up the daughter of two educators, I was nurtured. I often say my dad was my biggest cheerleader and my mom was my coach. When I expressed that I wanted to be a doctor, they counseled me to "get around" doctors so that I could see what they do. When it came time to go to college, I worked really hard, and I was one of five students during my junior year in college to be accepted into the Early Selection Program between Oakwood University and Loma Linda University School of Medicine. I graduated with honors.

Fast forward, and it was my last year of medical school when I was reacquainted with a former classmate of mine from Oakwood—Wendell McMillan II. I remember thinking back to biochemistry class when I first saw this quiet, good-looking man sitting in the row next to the periodic table and how I decided to change my seat to sit next to him so I could, "find out his story." Well, needless to say that initial conversation came full circle June 2, 2002.

Our union brought into the world two beautiful children. Now, it wasn't easy. They were both high-risk pregnancies. But they were both worth every minute of bed rest and progesterone injections. They keep me on my toes by how smart they are. They are kind and funny, and I like hanging with them.

After completing residency I went into the "real world" and joined a private practice. At this time, I heard about a new technology that could help my precision with minimally invasive surgeries. As a young attending physician at a community hospital, I took it upon myself to became certified in the use of the DiVinci Robotic Operating System. I was the only GYN using a million-dollar machine on a weekly basis, bringing in over $80K in revenue within the first six months of its use.

Now, I have a question for you. Is it okay if I share my real story with you?

Would you agree that there are some days in your life that you will never forget? That day for me is April 2, 2009. It started out as any regular call day. I had four minor cases lined up for the OR. I remember I pulled into my parking spot in the physician's parking lot, went in, and met my first patient in the pre-op area. It was a good OR day. My cases were on time, and my OR team was in rhythm. As I was walking out to talk to patient number 3's family, one of the OR nurses caught up with me and said, "Hey, Doc, before you go to L&D after this last case, I need you to see me." I said okay, but I noted that she paused and said it again with emphasis. "Make sure you see *me*."

Well, this didn't seem out of the ordinary, because I was always asked to give off-the-record consults. I finished my last case and found Tracey. She then led me into the pediatric holding area in the pre-op area and there sitting in the rocking chair was my husband. My first thought was, "How sweet, you came to have lunch with me." Then I really *looked* at his face. My next thought was, "Oh Lord, who in his family just died?" (You see, unfortunately his family was experiencing a string of losses around this same time.)

I remember him lovingly putting his arm around my waist and drawing me in to sit on his knee as he began to tell me that they are not sure what happened, they don't know if it was a heart attack or another stroke, but my dad didn't make it.

At that moment, I believe I felt the coldness of death totally engulf my body. I began to hit my husband and tell him he was lying. My dad was fine. "He was *fine*!" I kept shouting. You see, I had just talked to my mother on my way into work that morning. We were coordinating Daddy's follow-up doctor's visits for when I was returning to Huntsville. He had suffered a stroke the month before and he was doing *fine*.

My curdling screams, which could be heard into the pre-op area, were so out of character for me that the anesthesiologist on call came in and asked me and my husband if I needed a sedative.

We buried my dad April 9, 2009. During the next five years, life would knock me down. We would bury my grandmother 10 months later. Three years after that, we would bury my grandfather. In the midst of our family losses, my brother would have some legal challenges, and my mother would develop a heart condition, and now I'm worrying all the time, waiting for the other shoe to drop.

And as the saying goes, the show must go on. So, I sat for my specialty boards twice, and guess what, I didn't pass. Now this didn't mean I was no longer a doctor. #Facts it was a goal I didn't achieve.

I didn't realize it at the time, but because of how I related to the world, I was developing an identity crisis. I know, I know. "What do you mean, an identity crisis?"

You see, I had identified myself at times as Norton and Linda's daughter. I remember sitting in my therapist's office unpacking the layers of my father's death and asking, "Can I still say I'm Norton and Linda's daughter?" I mean, he was gone.

I also didn't realize that because I was grieving not passing my specialty boards, I was experiencing the same thing. Could I still say I was an OBGYN? Guess what? Yes, I could. I still had my medical degree, and I still had my certificates of completion from two residency programs for obstetrics and gynecology. I still had my certification for operating the DiVinci robotic machine for minimally invasive laparoscopic surgery.

Well, guess what I did? I did some healing, left the world of traditional obstetrics and gynecology, and discovered a different way to give my genius to the world.

I'm Dr. LaKeischa, integrative GYN and hormone specialist. I help ambitious women suffering with depleting hormones. Through my concierge practice, speaking circuit, and book, I help you get your hormones balanced, regain mental sharpness, and have energy to last the entire day. You can become a balanced beauty (#balancedbeauties) by following me on all social media platforms @drlakeischamd. Now, let's get started.

Chapter 1

WHERE ARE YOU ON THE HORMONE SEESAW?

Has your cycle changed or stopped?

Are you one of the lucky ones who doesn't have to stock up on "feminine hygiene products" anymore? If you are still having your period, I'm going to let you in on a little secret. The truth is your hormones start changing way before you go into menopause. It's called perimenopause. This is when you start seeing changes either in the characteristics in the flow of your cycle or changes in the timing of your cycle. What do I mean? Your periods can start getting heavier or lighter. The other change can be your periods can start coming closer together or farther apart.

Are you starting to have symptoms that say your hormones are depleting?

We have all heard the stories about someone breaking out in the infamous sweat in the middle of nowhere. It wells up from their belly, it seems, and goes all the way to the top of their head, and they feel as if they are on fire. Well, not everyone is going to exhibit those symptoms. I often say, "Not everyone's body reads the textbooks." There are other symptoms that can give you clues that your hormone levels are dropping. Do you want to know what they are? Are you starting to have what seem to be "more yeast infections" than you used to? Is sex becoming more painful? Is your body feeling different and you can't seem to figure out how to feel "your normal" again?

Do you still have your sexy?

I don't know about you, but I remember hearing that women hit their sexual peak in their 40s. If you don't mind, may I share something with you? I fear I have to admit I had a rude awakening when I didn't experience that. What was wrong? Why didn't I still have my sexy? Why didn't I want to have sex as much as I did before we had kids? What was wrong with me? Am I preaching to the choir?

Sleep. Are you getting any?

Is it getting harder for you to get to sleep? Is it because you get a second wind in the evening or your brain just doesn't seem to shut off? Are you able to get to sleep but now you find yourself waking up at 3am every morning and looking at the clock and not going back to sleep until 5am? Next thing you know, that dog-gone alarm is going off, and you have to start your day. You muster up the strength to get out of bed, but you're worried because you have that big meeting today and you need to be mentally sharp for your presentation.

Do you wake up in a body you don't recognize?

You have gotten everybody else off for the morning, and now you go to get dressed. You reach for your power outfit because at least you'll look like the powerful c-suite exec you are. Oh no, wait a minute. It doesn't quite fit the way it used to. You go to stand in front of the mirror and starring back at you is a figure you don't recognize. How did you wake up in a body you don't even know anymore?

Is everybody getting on your last nerve?

"Yes, I heard you!"

"Why did she send me an email about this project again?"

"I drove all the way over here. Why didn't you tell me cheer practice was changed?"

"No, you can't have the car tonight?"

Really? He wants sex tonight? Sigh. I hope I didn't say that out loud.

Does it seem as if you only have one nerve left and *everybody* seems to be dancing all over it? You say to yourself, "What is going on? I used to be able to let things roll off of me. I was tough. Nothing came my way that I couldn't handle, but now I get overwhelmed so easily and I feel myself….just…shutting…down."

Are you worried you might have early-onset dementia?

Have you ever walked into a room and wondered, "Now, why did I come in here again?" Of course, I'm not saying that this is not normal. It happens to everyone every once in a while. However, there's a difference between that and not feeling as sharp as you used to be. And this feeling is impacting your life. You are starting to shrink in all areas of your life and not be as impactful as you once were.

SEX HORMONE CHECKLIST

	Yes	No
Are you still having a cycle?		
Has your cycle changed?		
Do you have brain fog?		
Do you have hot flashes?		
Do you have night sweats?		
Do you have vaginal dryness?		
Do you have a lot of yeast infections?		
Do you have problems falling asleep?		
Do you have problems staying asleep?		
If you answered yes to the sleep questions, is this new?		
Do you have breast tenderness right before your cycle?		

Do you get very irritated right before
your cycle starts?

Do you have cravings for certain foods
right before your cycle?

Do you have unexplained weight gain?

Do you have low sex drive?

Note: if you answered yes to any of these questions,
schedule your free strategy session with me at
www.talkhormones.com.

Chapter 2

WHAT IS A HORMONE?

A hormone is a molecule our body makes in one area, and it has influence or causes a reaction in another area of our body. It's that simple. An example of a hormone is Vitamin D. Yes, Vitamin D. It is made in the liver, and then it travels to our bones to help keep them strong.

Are hormones good or bad for me?

Hormones are not inherently good or bad. When they are made, they are made by one organ system, and then they travel through the bloodstream to another organ system and tell them what they are supposed to do. You should not administer hormones without the supervision of a physician. They know how to determine the correct dosing for your body and how to adjust the dosing as your body changes.

Addressing the pink elephant in the room—the WHI study

The reason women ask the question about hormones being bad for them is because of the WHI (Women's Health Initiative) study that came out in 2002. I'll never forget finding out about this study. It was my first day of residency, and my program director came into morning report frantic, stating that a copy of the report was delivered to her home by Federal Express. The next thing I knew, women were coming into our clinic scared, confused, and demanding to be taken off of their hormones. Looking back over the study as well as what we as physicians did in response to that study, I have come to some realizations I would like to share.

The reason that the study was done in the first place is that scientists realized that women in their childbearing ages didn't have heart attacks like men. The incidence of women having heart attacks seemed to increase when they went into menopause. It was speculated that this was due to the amount of estrogen and progesterone we have in our bodies when we are in our reproductive years. So why not give women who have had a heart attack estrogen and progesterone and see if we can stop them from having another heart attack.

The realizations I have come to are that:

1. We never fully explained the reason for the study. They looked at women 63 years or older who had had a known cardiovascular event and they wanted to prevent a second event.

2. We failed to have identify the forms of the hormones that were used. They were synthetic and made from horse urine.

3. We didn't have follow-up conversations about what this meant for women just starting to have hormone changes and didn't have a history of a heart attack.

4. We didn't start having the conversation about what we are learning about bio-identical hormones and how they can really change the landscape of your health

5. We didn't have the conversation about the big C: cancer.

Chapter 3

WHAT ARE THE BIG THREE SEX HORMONES AND WHAT DO THEY DO?

**Estrogen, progesterone, and testosterone—
what are they?**

What are the big three sex hormones? They are estrogen, progesterone, and testosterone. They all have their individual roles, and they also work together.

Before we talk about function, let's talk about location. For the purposes of this book, we will keep it very simple. Estrogen, progesterone, and testosterone mainly come from the ovaries. The ovaries respond to a signal that comes from the brain (the pituitary gland) called FSH (follicle stimulating hormone). This tells the ovaries it's time to make an egg. The ovaries hear this signal, they say okay, and they start recruiting an egg by increasing the levels of estrogen and progesterone. Once the brain receives a feedback signal that the ovaries hear it, then it stops increasing the level of FSH.

A way to assess if your hormones are starting to wane is by knowing what they do when the levels are optimal. I'm able to start assessing this by asking about a woman's cycle. Over the years, as a result of this process, I have come to some realizations. May I share those realizations with you?

As the doctor, I am speaking a different language from you, and I am going to give you the ability to translate what your doctor is saying so he or she will be better able to help you.

When your doctor asks, "Do you have a regular period?" they want to know how long it is between the first day you see your period to the next first day you see your period. This is not when you give how many days the flow last. Counting 28, 30, or 32 days between day 1 and the next day 1 is a normal cycle. This tells the doctor a lot of information, because when your interval starts changing, this is a sign that there is a change in the level of hormones you were once producing.

Let me help you pull this together. During the various phases of our lives, our hormones are at different levels, and the result of these varying levels show up in different ways.

Sex hormones, your period, and having a baby

You remember "the talk." "Your body is going to be changing, and you are going to start feeling things." (In my best Chandler Bing voice) Could you and the adult who had that conversation with you *be* any more uncomfortable? ☺ As you know, your sex hormones help with the development of your breasts, growing hair on your body (which can be a pain to manage), and the development of certain centers in your brain. As you move on in life from your late teens to young adulthood, you have moved from novice to amateur to pro in dealing with your period. You know when it's going to come. You know how many pads or tampons you use. You know to have that special pair of jeans that fit during "that time of the month" and which clothes are the "don't even take me off the hanger" clothes.

Can I give you a way to understand why you are able to become a pro at managing your period? Think of your period this way. Estrogen is in charge of making the grass grow tall. This is the uterine lining getting thick and ready for a fertilized egg to come and grow. Progesterone is in charge of mowing the grass. Depending on how high the grass is will determine how heavy the flow.

When there is a signal that there was no fertilized egg this month, progesterone comes and mows the lawn. This is your cycle every 28/30/32 days, and you start learning the routine and get very good at managing it and how it affects your life.

Now how does testosterone play into all of this? At this time, as far as we know, testosterone plays a huge role in our libido—our desire to have sex. Testosterone also helps to retain lean muscle and plays a role in our metabolism. I know, some of you are saying, "I don't want to look like no man!" Your natural levels of testosterone do not allow for that. Testosterone also helps with our brain health. It helps our neurotransmitters, which need to be at certain levels to help with focus. There are also anti-inflammatory properties that testosterone has.

The change

I don't know about you, but growing up, I always only heard about a woman going through "the change." It wasn't until I was a physician that I started understanding and hearing the term perimenopause (around menopause). Perimenopause can be described as a time in your life where you are starting to experience depletion in your hormones but you are still having your period. I like the emerging term of Testosterone Deficiency Syndrome (TDS). Yes, I hear you. "Wait? This is for real? You mean I'm not going crazy?" No, you are not. See, this is the part of "the talk" we have been missing. It's not our mothers' fault. There was no name for it back then. Everybody just powered through. Were you told that it's just the way life is? That you are just getting older? Welcome to the other side.

I can remember reading a story about another physician who shared in her book her story about how she was starting to gain weight, not wanting to have sex with her husband, and was feeling depressed. She went to her own primary care doctor, and they told her she was just "getting older." They even told her she was experiencing some depression, and they wanted to start her on an anti-depressant. Well, she refused. She knew there was something wrong with her. She began to research and started understanding TDS. She started bio-identical hormone therapy, and she started feeling so much better!

Part of the empowerment you have now is understanding that as adolescence and childbearing phases are on a continuum, so is perimenopause (TDS) and menopause. The empowerment is that you now can have a guide that will help you navigate the changes of this phase of life. In my opinion, in the past, we have looked at menopause as a single event. And I can see how that comes about. We have definitions in medicine, which keeps order. The textbook classification of menopause is when you have 12 consecutive months without a period. It does not have to be accompanied by hot flashes, night sweats, and significant vaginal dryness.

Like I mentioned in Chapter 1, if you are like me, you remember as a young girl growing up seeing women all of a sudden have beads of sweat break out across their forehead and start dripping down their face. Some of them would start fanning feverishly, and you may hear another woman nearby whisper, "She's going through the change." "The change?" What was that? Was it something you caught? Was it something you had to go through? Was it avoidable?

What did this mean? Was that lady going to die soon? Well, no, not necessarily physically, but there were parts of her "self" that were "dying." This book is to stop the whispers and start the clear conversation about how your hormones start depleting as you are moving toward menopause. The second part of that conversation is how with the advent of research and medicine, you can survive the next phase of your hormone evolution and thrive.

The change in the levels of estrogen and progesterone are seen by the decrease in fertility. She wasn't having anymore babies. The decrease in estrogen, progesterone, and testosterone can also be involved in temperature regulation. This comes in the form of hot flashes and night sweats.

Estrogen also keeps the vagina healthy. When estrogen starts dropping, the vagina begins to get dry. Estrogen also helps keep the collagen in our skin strong and conditioned. This helps to reduce smile and frown lines (wrinkles). Estrogen also keeps the bladder healthy. Wait what did I just say? Yes, that's right. Those new symptoms of urinary incontinence could be from decreasing estrogen. Think of the vagina as a room. The entrance is the outside of the vagina. The ceiling is the bladder, the floor is the rectum, and the back wall is the cervix leading to the uterus. When you are young and there is plenty of estrogen on board, the vagina has hills and valleys. That is healthy tissue. As you get older and the levels of estrogen start to decrease, those hills and valleys turn in to an ice-skating rink. Now imagine, this surface now is scratchy like burlap wool. That is irritating, isn't it? This is irritating to the ceiling and thus causes the bladder to become spastic, thus causing you to feel like you have a UTI.

Progesterone is the hormone that keeps you feeling balanced. It gives you a nice big hug and helps you turn your brain off at night so you can get good restorative sleep. Progesterone also gives some fuel to the adrenal glands to help with dealing with stress (we'll come back to this).

Testosterone is the hormone that makes you want to have sex, but it is also implicated in your mood, motivation, and focus. It also helps you to burn fat and retain lean muscle. No, testosterone will not make you get bulky like a man. Testosterone is also showing protective effects on breast tissue (I am not saying it will totally prevent breast cancer).

Together, estrogen and testosterone show protective effects on bone health. When used with Vitamin D supplementation, it can help with building bone and help decrease your risk for developing osteopenia and osteoporosis.

Chapter 4

THE BIG THREE SEX HORMONES AND HOW THEY HELP YOU RUN EFFICIENTLY

The sex hormones don't just run the show by themselves. They have other organ systems that help you run efficiently. The other two systems that do this are the adrenal glands and the thyroid gland. Once again, before we talk about function, let's talk about location. The adrenal glands sit on top of the kidneys like little berets. The thyroid gland sits in the front of the throat area. These two gland systems are also controlled by the pituitary gland located in the brain. (I don't know if you see the pattern yet, but the pituitary is the conductor, and everybody has to answer to it).

I want you to think of yourself as a car. The sex hormones are the computer system, the adrenal glands are your engine, and your thyroid gland is the gas pedal.

Adrenal glands

The adrenal glands are the engine in your car. They produce your stress hormones—cortisol, epinephrine, norepinephrine, and adrenaline—to help you get through your day or help keep you alive. You've heard a car change gears, right? When the car is shifting, it is accommodating the needs of the car. When your body sends a signal that it needs help dealing with stress or is in danger, your adrenal glands kick in. Your adrenal glands protect you from danger. You've heard of the fight or flight pathway in your body? This is one of the adrenal's main jobs. When you swerve and miss that car and avoid that car accident and you feel that fire sensation flare up from your core, that was the adrenals doing what they were supposed to do—help you survive. The problem comes when the engine gets stuck in second gear. It cannot sustain this demand long term.

Thyroid gland

The thyroid gland is the gas pedal in your car. Pushing
the gas pedal helps you have energy, increases your metabolism, regulates your temperature, helps keep your
intestinal health regular, and keeps your skin and hair
healthy. This occurs when TSH (thyroid stimulating
hormone), which comes from the brain, tells the thyroid
gland it's time to make thyroid hormone. The gland hears
the pituitary and makes two forms: Free T4 and Free T3.
Free T4 is known as the inactive form of the hormone,
and Free T3 is known as the active form. I tell patients
to think of it this way—Free T4 is like the right key fit-
ting in the right lock. Free T3 is like turning that key in
the lock. Free T4 is converted into Free T3 throughout
the body. When the thyroid gland is not working well,
you feel tired or can hit an energy slump during the day.
When you exercise, you can't seem to lose weight. You
feel cold when everyone else is comfortable, or you have
cold hands and feet. You become constipated very easily.
You have dry skin outside of winter. And the big one—
your crown (your hair) is now thinning, and you are
drawing on your eyebrows because they are not growing
all the way to the edge of your eye line like they used to.

Sex hormones

The sex hormones are the computer system that helps your car run smoothly. When your sex hormones are balanced, your mood is even. You get good, restorative sleep. You are able to check items off of your "to do" list because you are motivated again. You are running the c-suite with ease because your brain is sharp. Your skin looks amazing. And guess what? You want to have sex!

In order for you to run smoothly all of these components have to be at peak performance. Now if the engine (adrenals) is idling in second gear, then it's going to start pulling on the computer system (sex hormones), and when you go to push on the gas pedal (thyroid), you won't be able to get the car to go.

When you make sure your engine (adrenals) is tuned up, then you won't strain the computer system (sex hormones), and when you go to push on the gas pedal (thyroid), you will be able to go, go, go! And when the system is working together how does this look? I'll say it again. You can get good, restorative sleep. You want to have sex. You can exercise and see the results again. People want to be around you. And because your mind is sharp again, you are rocking the c-suite with ease!

Let's check in on your adrenal and thyroid health before we go on.

	Yes	No
Adrenal health		
Do you feel rested when you wake up in the mornings?		
Do you have an energy slump during the day?		
Do you get a second wind in the evening?		
Do you feel wired but tired?		
Thyroid health		
Do you feel you have low energy all day?		
Do you have cold hands and/or cold feet?		
Do you have constipation?		
Do you have brain fog?		
Do you have dry skin outside of winter?		

Do you have thinning hair?

Do your eyebrows not grow all the way
to the edge of the outer eyeline?

Note: If you answered yes to any of these questions,
schedule your free strategy session with me at
www.talkhormones.com

Chapter 5

HOW DO YOU GET THE HELP YOU NEED?

You should be seeing your OB-GYN at least once a year. This is called your Well Woman Exam (WWE). This is important for breast and pelvic health assessment. Just as a reminder, it's at this visit that you get a breast exam and referral for a mammogram. You get a pap smear done along with possible HPV testing (your OB-GYN will know who gets that testing and how often). You also get a pelvic exam to make sure there are no large tumors growing in the pelvis. This is the exam where, depending on your age, you will get referrals for other important screening test like a DEXA scan as well as reminders to talk to your primary care doctor about your need for colonoscopy referral and a vaccination schedule.

At this visit, you can start telling your doctor the changes you are experiencing. Let them know if you are having hot flashes, night sweats, or vaginal dryness that is making sex uncomfortable. Hell, do you even want to have sex anymore? Let them know if you are now having weight gain despite assessing your diet and improving your exercise plan. Let them know if you are now not able to handle the stressors of life. Let them know if you can't sleep, or if you are not on top of your game at work and you need help. Do you have to wait for this visit? No! You can make an appointment at anytime to see your doctor and start a conversation.

I hear you. You are screaming at me, "What if my doctor doesn't think anything is wrong with me? What if they just tell me to eat less and exercise more? What if they say, 'Oh you just need to get more sleep.' What if they tell me I need an anti-depressant or anti-anxiety medication to deal with the stress? What if they tell me that I am just getting old and that's just life?"

If these answers are okay for you, then fine, but if you are shaking your head, then find another doctor who will listen to you and become a partner in helping you to figure out what is best for you.

What else do you need to look at besides just your symptoms? There are a variety of labs that can help look at the different systems we talked about in Chapter 4. This information can be used in concert with your symptoms to help devise a plan for you.

- For the sex hormones: Estradiol, Estrone, Progesterone, Testosterone (free and total), FSH

- For thyroid: TSH, Free T4, Free T3, Thyroid Antibodies, Reverse T3

- For adrenals: DHEA-S, Saliva Cortisol Test

Chapter 6

KNOW WHAT IS AVAILABLE FOR YOU IN ORDER TO GET BALANCED

Going back to the pink elephant in the room—the WHI study. Remember I said that we needed to start a conversation about what is available now and how it is different? Bio-identical hormones are here. What are bio-identical hormones? These are hormones that look just like what your body makes. Some of their components come from plants, and they are made in a laboratory. Because they are bio-identical, your body recognizes them and says, "Hey, I know what this is," and it breaks it down and utilizes it the way it should. I get the question all the time, "What can I do to help my body to produce more hormones?" The general answer is there is very little you can do to increase your own production of hormones after a certain age. (Because each person is unique, once you work with a doctor and you tell them your specifics, they can customize a plan for you).

Now that you know what bio-identical hormones are. What form do they come in? There is pellet therapy and cream therapy. Pellets are made by a compounding pharmacy. This specialized pharmacy can make customized dosing for individuals, unlike a commercial pharmacy, which can only distribute pre-made dosing that comes from a pharmaceutical supplier.

The pellet insertion is done in an office setting. You are given a numbing agent like lidocaine (just like when you go to the dentist). This is placed in the hip area. Once you are numb, a stab incision is made, and then the trocar is placed into the hip through the incision into an area of fatty tissue. The pellets are then deployed into that fatty pocket. The skin is sealed by either steri-strips or skin glue. The testosterone pellet is about the size of a Tylenol capsule, and an estrogen pellet is about the fourth of that size.

Creams are also a way to deploy bio-identical hormone therapy to the body. Depending on your doctor, they will either split the estrogen and testosterone prescriptions or they will write them as a combination. The creams usually come in a deodorant type of dispenser. You will have instructions on how many clicks to use per day. I usually tell my patients to use the dispenser to apply the cream. The creams are very rich, so it may seem like it takes a long time for them to completely absorb into the skin. The compounded creams do not transfer to others with whom you come in contact, so don't worry.

I am often asked which method is better. It depends on the patient and their lifestyle and desires. Let me explain. The pellets are what I call "set it and forget it." Once they are in, they are in. You cannot go and retrieve them. The level of hormones available through pellets tends to be consistent once they reach their peak levels. The creams can tend to not give as even and steady amount because it depends on the end user—you. You have to put it on every day and ideally at the same time every day. Some (depending on your starting hormone levels) will require multiple applications a day. Now, if you are a very disciplined person and you can add creams into your life regimen, then that is wonderful! However, if you are not that confident in your ability to be the captain of your hormone ship, then set it and forget it is probably the course for you.

There is another option for oral consumption. This is not utilized often for estrogen because it is very difficult to balance the estrogen ratio (E1/E2). There is no oral formulation for testosterone. Progesterone is the exception. Progesterone can come in both cream and capsule form. There is discussion of whether or not the oral form of progesterone can more accurately show increases in the blood levels over the cream formulations.

The reason topical and pellet preparations are preferred methods for dispensing bio-identical is because they avoid first-pass metabolism. No need to get nervous. This simply means they don't have to go through the liver to be processed. This way, the liver doesn't have to work so hard in helping to break the hormones down and get the various components to where they need to go.

Remember that not only do we need to balance the sex hormones, we also need to take care of the adrenal gland (the engine) and the thyroid gland (the gas pedal).

Let's talk about how we tune up the engine. We tune up the engine (adrenals) by giving them the building blocks they need so they can make the stress hormones as needed and stop stealing from the computer system (sex hormones). Here is where you can give your body the right fuel and you can help make more of these types of hormones. A good adrenal support vitamin can give the adrenals the building blocks they need so that they can make the stress hormones that are needed in various situations. You should look for look for Rhodiola and ashwagandha in a good adrenal support supplement. An amino acid called L-theanine can also help give support to the adrenals.

The next component we need to make sure is taken care of is the gas pedal (thyroid gland). When the thyroid gland is optimal, then when you push on the gas pedal and need to increase your metabolism, increase your internal temperature, stay regular, keep your skin and hair conditioned, and have enough energy to make it to the finish line of your days, there is nothing to it. Again, here is where you can get a good thyroid support vitamin, and it can help the thyroid convert Free T4 into Free T3 more efficiently and have more of the active form of the thyroid hormone available. There are vitamins and minerals that can help your body be as efficient as possible with the conversion of Free T4 to Free T3, including selenium, iodine Vitamin B12, and Vitamin C. The other key to helping the thyroid function at its best is having a healthy gut. What does this mean? When our gut (intestines) have not been treated very kindly over the years with our food choices, there can be inflammation in the gut that prevents the most effective absorption of the fuel we take in through our food. When this happens, we don't convert Free T4 into Free T3. It goes to another pathway that makes a molecule called Reverse T3. This cannot be utilized as well to help create energy, regulate temperature, and optimize skin health. Higher levels of Reverse T3 mean that you not only need a supplement to help convert Free T4 to Free T3, but you also need to work on your gut health.

Chapter 7

UNDERSTAND HOW STRESS AFFECTS YOUR HORMONES

When we think of how our bodies work in the simplest way, we can distill our understanding down to this simple analogy. The body only wants to survive or have sex, have fun, and reproduce. Take a moment and think about this. You are driving on the freeway going just slightly over the speed limit because you were doing the two-step shuffle this morning (that dog-gone brain fog got you again) and it took you longer to get out of the house. You know you'll be on time if everybody on the freeway cooperates with your plans this morning and just stays in their lanes. Well wouldn't you know it, there is that one person who doesn't see you in their blind spot. They are changing into your lane, matching you at speed, and in order to avoid the damage to the passenger's side of your car, days of body shop repairs, and all the trimmings that go along with a high-speed collision, you *slam* on your breaks just in the nick of time! And now you feel it—that flare of fire in the center of your core. Your breathing increases, your heart is beating fast, and your hands are steadying the wheel but you still feel the micro tremors like aftershocks flowing through your fingers. The adrenal glands did what they needed to do in order to help you survive.

Now, think of this—not being able to meet that office deadline. There she goes again, the one person on the team you manage at work is making you look bad to the CEO again. It's time for college admissions for your oldest, your middle child needs braces, and the youngest wants to start piano lessons, and you just can't figure out how to get it all done. All of these scenarios are producing the same flare of fire in the center of your core. Your adrenal glands think they need to produce the same level of stress hormones as when you almost lost your life in that near-miss car accident. This is what stuck in second gear looks like. Your engine is revving. An engine revving in one gear will break down after a while.

So what does the body do to try and help the engine (adrenal glands)? It starts seeing who can spare some resources. It looks around and goes, "Oh yeah, the computer system (sex hormones) shares a common pathway with me." What does this mean? There is a parent molecule that likes to go down the sex hormone pathway or the stress hormone pathway. When the body is stressed, it opts to save you. I mean why have sex, have fun, and reproduce when you just need to survive?

The other component that is affected when there is a stress signal is the gas pedal. There are connections noted in the literature that show that when the body receives a stress signal, the connection with the hypothalamic-pituitary adrenal (HPA) axis is dampened. This is how the brain sends signals to various places in our body. It is at this level that the pituitary sends a message to the thyroid gland that says, "Hey, you need to make more thyroid hormone," and in turn, it gets feedback from the thyroid that says, "Thanks, I heard you." This happens when the levels of Free T4 and Free T3 increase. When you get a stress signal in the body, there can be a dampening of the signal from the brain to the thyroid gland, so the gland doesn't make as much hormone as it used to or needs to. In turn, what happens?

You try to step on the gas to increase your metabolism, increase your temperature, make sure your gut can eliminate the waste, and make sure your hair and skin are healthy, but nothing. And the ultimate—you don't have the energy to cross the finish line to make it through your days. And you just can't!

Chapter 8

BALANCING YOUR HORMONES HELPS YOU FIND YOURSELF AGAIN

For some time now, you have been feeling as if you have been walking sideways, am I right? I know how you feel. I've felt the same way. You know what I found? Once I balanced my hormones, I began to feel better.

Is it okay if I share a vulnerable moment with you? I see you nodding yes, so here goes. In the spring of 2019, I was the heaviest I had ever weighed in my life. I was 197 pounds. My blood pressure was in the 170s/110s. I knew I had to do something. In 2017, my internist left the practice I was going to, and my OB-GYN had retired. I had not been to a doctor in a year. In May of 2019, I found an internist and an OB-GYN. I worked on getting my hormones balanced, and I did some biohacking to work on getting my weight off. While in this process, I partnered with a nutritionist, and she helped me with my gut health and I started exercising again. By September 2019, I had lost 23 pounds. I am exercising again on a regular basis, my hormones are balanced (yes, I use bio-identical hormones, and when you become a #balancedbeauty I'll share more of my story ☺), I have regained mental sharpness, and I feel beautiful and vital again.

What is another way to look at this? I began to feel like myself again. My family began to like me again. I remember my son saying to me one time, "Mommy you're not yelling as much anymore. Your voice doesn't have that rapid beat to it anymore. It has a slower beat to it." Isn't that something when your energy waves are different?

My energy levels increased significantly. I wasn't dragging across the finish line anymore at the end of the day. I was getting sleep again! I was waking up feeling rested and ready to face the day. I was able to tolerate life's stressors a little better. I began to care about myself and make sure my cup was full so that I could pour into others. My brain fog was gone! I could think clearly again. I felt beautiful again, and my zest for life was renewed.

Wouldn't it be great to feel good again? Wouldn't it feel good to like who you are again? Wouldn't it be just amazing to have more energy? Wouldn't you feel like you could conquer the world if you got better sleep? Wouldn't you love to see the mental sharpness of that ambitious woman you know you are return? Wouldn't you jump at the chance to feel beautiful and vital?

Chapter 9

HOW DO YOU SURVIVE PERIMENOPAUSE AND MENOPAUSE?

Have a real conversation with yourself, and those in your circle.

It's time to have some real conversations with yourself, your family and friends. What do I mean by this? Start with yourself. Be honest with yourself and admit there is something wrong. Admit to yourself, "Yes, I did wake up in a body I don't recognize. Everyone is getting on my last nerve, and I feel as if I'm going crazy."

Next, open up to your partner. Talk about how you are feeling. Tell them that you are having a problem and you need their help to solve it. Tell them that you don't feel like yourself anymore. Tell them you don't have the energy to get through the day and you know this is not normal. Even though they may already know, still tell them that you are not sleeping well. Let them know you feel as if you haven't slept at all the night before because your brain never turned off. Or tell them that you woke up and had to turn on the fan and strip because you were hot and bothered. But not because you wanted to have sex—far from it. You were having a hot flash or a night sweat. Tell them that you don't have the reserve to handle the slightest stress anymore and you feel if one more person asks you to do another thing you just might explode. Take them inside your brain and show them how you feel now that the lights don't turn all the way on anymore, and that means you are not as mentally sharp as you used to be. And then probably the hardest conversation to have is explaining to your partner how you don't want to have sex anymore. Yes, this one is difficult for men to grasp. The way I help men understand this concept is that women's sex organ is between their ears. Your brain is where 90 percent of your libido lies. If the HPA axis is not working and your hormone levels are decreasing, you don't have a desire to have sex.

The next stop in your circle is your family. Listen to your children. And listen to their non-verbal communication as much as you listen to their verbal. Create a safe space where they can feel comfortable giving you their observations of you as a person. This will also lay the groundwork for developing a long-term relationship outside of the parent-child relationship as they grow into an adult and your relationship changes focus to an adult-adult relationship.

Now, I know you have some girlfriends who can help you check in. Those girlfriends who help you remember you were a person first before you were so-and-so's wife and so-and-so's mother. You know who I'm taking about. She's that girlfriend who shares with you the great deal she found at your favorite store as you both escape your worlds over a glass of wine, sitting on her back porch, daring anyone to call your name. Go to her and ask her, "Can I check in?" Tell her you don't feel like yourself anymore and you need someone who is going to be honest with you and help you figure out what is wrong and how you can get back to yourself.

And just like how she shares the latest store deals with you, she just so happens to have heard about perimenopause and menopause and how you don't have to just "power through it." There are treatments out there to help women nowadays. You don't have to suffer in silence like your mother and grandmother did.

Continue the conversation with your doctor

Once you have done your field research on *you*, now it's time to continue the conversation with your doctor. Make a list of symptoms that you have been having and a timeline for those symptoms. Also add a list of questions that you want to have answered. This helps to keep the conversation flowing and on track. Check in with yourself and see if you feel heard by your doctor. Then listen to your doctor's assessment of your symptoms and plan of action. Make sure you understand their recommendations for the course of action. Ask them how their plan will help to ameliorate or improve your symptoms, and understand possible side effects. If their recommendations and expectations are not what you are seeking, then find another doctor. This may not be the right fit for either of you, and that's okay.

Once you have found the right physician for you, know that this is a marathon. This is not a sprint. You didn't get to this point overnight, and there is no magic potion to restore you to balance overnight. It may take adjustments in the dosing of your bio-identical hormone therapy (BHRT) regimen before you get total relief of your symptoms. It may also take a multi-system approach to get you feeling balanced. What do I mean by that? You may need your thyroid balanced. Your adrenals may need to be supported. You may need to do a gut cleanse. So be patient. Give yourself grace on this path to becoming balanced again.

Continue to add tools to your life to help you stay balanced

Alright! You have your hormones on board. Now what? It's time to add more tools to your survival guide. I tell patients all the time, it's not only what you put on the inside that counts, but it's other synergistic therapies and life changes that can help you not only survive but thrive through perimenopause and menopause.

Therapy/life coaching/mentors/tribes

One of the big tools I recommend you having is a therapist and/or life coach. Now that you have mental sharpness again, you can have clarity of thought. I know you are asking why I said therapist and/or life coach? Well, sometimes you may need one or both.

A life coach can help you organize your life and give you specific tools you can use to tackle various situations in your world. This can be viewed as them helping you do the heavy lifting of acknowledging certain patterns exist in your life and the way you normally try to resolve them is not working for you.

A therapist can do the same healing work as a life coach in helping you acknowledge patterns and helping you to break free of destructive patterns, but they can go a little deeper and diagnosis possible mental health illnesses that need to be treated in order for you to have your breakthrough.

Can I share something with you? I have seen a therapist. Yes, you read that right. And you know what? It has been one of the best things I have ever done. Therapy helped me at the most difficult times in my life, and I often go back for what I call "tune ups." We are constantly evolving, and having these individuals in your life does something big for you. In my opinion, this helps us take that "S" off our chest, and we let ourselves off the hook in trying to be superwoman all the time. For some of us, therapy/life coaching helps create some necessary boundaries. Therapy to me is the same as when the airline attendant is going through the safety instructions on a plane and they tell you to "put your mask on first before helping anybody else." Do you know why they tell you to do that? Because you can't help anybody if you are passed out. Therapy helps you help others.

I have also had a life coach. I needed her because I was at a point in my life I didn't know what was next. I realized that for a very long time, my course to get to the goal of being a doctor was always mapped out. I have never had to do that myself. Using her gave me such a breakthrough in how to bring to the forefront a goal I had and make it crystal clear. Developing this skill has helped me learn how to make decisions very quickly because I know whether or not it is supporting a goal I am working to accomplish.

Mentorship is not only for people in business. You can have a mentor for any area of your life. And guess what? In this wonderful age of technology, you can have a virtual mentor. If you find someone online with whom you connect because their message is resonating with you, continue to follow them. Get whatever content they are putting out there. Then, if you are able to see them live, *do it*! There is something about sharing the same oxygen space and feeling the energy of like-minded people. It is infectious! I often recall for other moms a time I went to a conference and there was another mother on stage sharing her story. I could relate to her because she was from the Maryland/Washington, DC/Virginia area. She was talking about how they as a family had set some structure on how many extracurricular activities their

55

three children could be involved in at one time. And the reason was twofold. If each child had been involved in more than one activity at a time, she would be on the 495 beltway all the time! (I could relate to that.) They also wanted to teach their children the value of commitment and staying with something until completion. This conference happened years ago, and I still remember that sage advice.

Find your tribe! Get around like-minded women who affirm you and push you at the same time. I once heard that every five years, you can project where you will be in life by the people with whom you associate and the books you read. Mindset is everything! This brain of yours is a beautiful and wonderful creation. Our brains were designed to work toward a goal. When we are actively in pursuit of a goal, our brain *loves* that. It works for you so that you can achieve it. I'm going to say it again but I'm going to say it how our grandmothers would have said it—birds of a feather flock together.

Acupuncture and meditation

Another therapy to add to your survival guide is one that can help decrease inflammation in your body—acupuncture therapy. For some of you, this can be something that you need more information about in order to understand how this can work as part of your survival guide.

Can I share another piece of my story with you? It wasn't until 2016 that I learned more about the benefits of acupuncture medicine. Acupuncture medicine is another way to help the body heal and stay in balance. I was able to interview an acupuncture therapist who was trained in traditional Chinese medicine. She shared with me the analogy that if you think of yourself in simple chemistry terms, you are a bunch of positive and negative charges that need to line up in the right way in order for the system to function at full capacity. Acupuncture does just that. It helps to unblock any channels that may be blocked by an external or internal trauma by helping the charges to line up correctly. This practice can help keep hormones balanced, recharge the adrenal glands, and support the thyroid.

I experienced first-hand how acupuncture therapy helped heal my adrenal glands. It was 2016, and I began working at a wellness center. This was the first time I had labs done on myself to see where my sex hormones, thyroid function, and adrenal glands were registering. I should not have been surprised when my testosterone was not even measurable and my DHEA-S was 37. I had already accepted that acupuncture would be a way I could help get and keep my body in balance. It was at my second acupuncture therapy session that I spoke with the therapist and shared that my adrenals really needed help and I had symptoms of adrenal fatigue. We agreed she would do a therapy targeted to supporting my adrenals.

During the session, there was a moment I felt as if someone opened the valve on the pressure cooker and released the pressure. At the end of the session, my therapist informed me that when she placed her needles in the area that supported adrenal health, that area became very red, so much that she waited a little to make sure I wasn't having a histamine release. Once she was reassured this was my body showing that it needed healing and help, she allowed the therapy to go to completion. Subsequently, she has helped to optimize my thyroid health and manage my ADHD symptoms.

Another tool that helps decrease inflammation is meditation, worship, or prayer. I am a person of faith, and here is where I have had to relinquish to my faith. You see, science won't always give hard evidence to support what some say is antidotal practices. I believe, seen, and experienced where mediation, a good praise session, or a whispered prayer has calmed fear, quieted anxiety, and removed doubt. How does this look on a physiological level? It can lower blood pressure, decrease heart rate, increase focus, allow increase blood flow to the gut, and influence gut health.

Find a quiet place and time where you can claim as yours for meditation. There is no right way. Just start. You may have to change some clutter on your calendar so that you can put *you* on the calendar. Make this a non-negotiable appointment. If you don't know how to start, there are apps or YouTube channels available for the novice to the more seasoned meditation student.

Exercise

The next tool I want to highlight is one that can become a keystone habit. Our bodies were made to move. I had the privilege of interviewing martial arts/certified yoga instructor Josh Cradock. He also holds a degree in kinesiology. We talked about the concept that our bodies were made to move. He informed me that in the world of fitness, sitting is the new smoking. What this means is that a sedentary lifestyle is as big a risk factor for cardiovascular disease as being a smoker. Exercise not only helps with the obvious benefits of initial weight loss and lifelong management of your weight. It also helps to decrease stress, which indirectly supports improvement in some of the areas that perimenopause and menopause start depleting.

I know, I know, I know. You are saying you don't have the time to exercise. I will challenge you on this one. Have you ever heard about exercise snacking? Yup, the concept is as simple as it sounds. McMaster University, University of British Columbia's Okanagan campus in Canada, published a study in the September 2018 issue of the *Journal of Applied Physiology, Nutrition and Metabolism*. The study was, "Do Stair Climbing Exercise 'Snacks' Improve Cardiorespiratory Fitness?"

In short, exercise snacking is doing some form of exercise, like walking up steps instead of taking the elevator, walking at your lunch break, or walking in the evenings. You can do this for only 10-minute intervals at least three times a day at least five days, no less than three days a week.

And what they found was that it did improve cardiorespiratory fitness along with an incidental finding of improved skeletal muscle strength.

For those who are a little more advance in their exercise commitments, there are programs that can help you find your metabolic equivalent task (MET). This is different from high-intensity training (HIT). This is how much energy you need to expend per unit of your body weight during one minute of rest. In other words, how much energy do *you* need to generate in order to burn fat. It's more individualized. For example, I need 13 METs a week if I want to lose or maintain my weight. You can go online and see how many METs a particular exercise done for a certain amount of time generates.

In my opinion, exercise is so important in ways that are obvious and in the intangibles. Here's what I mean. I believe exercise is a keystone habit. I was introduced to the concept of a keystone habit by former head coach of the Indianapolis Colts, Tony Dungy. I heard him being interviewed on a podcast several years ago, and he was talking about how the defensive linemen coaching staff work with the players to develop plays. He went on to say that there were some foundational movements that the players had to get down first. These movements are very basic. They are even boring. They are not movements that would make the highlight reels. But they are movements that create muscle memory on which the coaching staff can now build to get the plays that make the highlight reel.

What does this mean for you and exercise? Exercise can become a keystone habit that leads to a domino effect of positive decisions you make in your life. For example, when I exercise, I drink more water. Because I drink more water, my brain is clearer. Because my brain is sharper, then I have clarity of though. When I have clarity of thought, I can even make better decisions about my food, money, business, and health. Do you see the dominos falling?

Here is the quick and dirty of how this works. When you exercise you release endorphins, those hormones in the brain we all know as the "feel good" hormones. Exercise can help support various neurotransmitter pathways that play a role in sleep, libido (sex drive), mood, focus, immune system health, and gut health.

Peri-menu-pause

Here is another tool to have to help you stay balanced. Learning how your gut health is the anchor to your hormone health. In the world of integrative medicine, it is believed that gut health is the root cause of so many imbalances in our hormone systems.

One way to make sure that your gut is taken care of is by making sure your water intake is adequate. Your cells *love* water. Water helps keep the cell membrane flexible so that it can maintain its integrity. Why does this seemingly random fact matter? Because the cell is the basis for tissues, and tissues make up organs, and organs make up organ systems. Drinking water can help with the conditioning of our skin and help slow down the signs of aging, and we can be #over40andfabulous. Of course, I get asked how much water should I drink? I am of the school of thought that you should be drinking half your body weight in ounces. (I know, I just saw your jaw drop). All you have to do is take your weight. Divide it in half, and that is how many ounces a day you should be drinking. Yes, you will be going to the bathroom, but once your body gets accustomed to having its optimal amount on board, you will feel the difference. Your energy levels will begin to increase, your brain fog will begin to lift, and your gut health will be better regulated.

We have all been told that sugar is bad. I would like to qualify by saying too much sugar yes. Sugar is pro-inflammatory, and I have been told by my patients that when they regulate the amount of excess sugar they consume, their hot flashes decrease dramatically.

The other discovery I have made is that when you have a healthy microbiome (population of bacteria), your gut is able to work efficiently in extracting the fuel sources from your foods. Your body does want some carbs because it uses the sugar molecule that carbs are made of because this is the most efficient way to produce energy.

An obstacle that can prevent the gut from being efficient is "leaky gut syndrome." This can occur when you have unknown food sensitivities and/or allergies. There are various tests that your doctor can order that can help you discover if you have any.

Food sensitivity testing can be assessed from a blood test looking at two immune system molecules: IgE, and IgG. IgE looks at true food allergies. This is the molecule that gives an immediate response from the immune system. The reaction is what we called the "wheels and flares." What I mean is that this shows up as a rash, immediate swelling, and itching (a full blown inflammatory response). Depending on how much of the molecule is stimulated, an individual that has this response to a food would need to carry around an epi pen.

IgG looks at food sensitivities. This is the molecule that makes a plan and waits. When they stimulate a response, the reaction is delayed. It can be 24, 48, or 72 hours later. And what type of reaction does it cause? You can have constipation, diarrhea, joint pain, swollen joints, headaches, foggy brain, or difficulty losing weight. And because these symptoms are delayed, you don't always connect feeling bad on Wednesday to something you ate on Sunday or Monday evening.

The other reason it is important to make sure that your gut is healthy is that you have receptors for thyroid hormones in your gut. If you recall, we talked about the various pathways that can utilize Free T4. If your gut is healthy, then Free T4 turns into the active form of the thyroid hormone, which is Free T3. This is what we talked about in Chapter 4. So now let's connect it. Free T4 cannot convert to Free T3, so it finds an easier pathway, and that is Reverse T3. This is how your gut tells on you. If your Reverse T3 is high, then you can make a connection to gut inflammation, and this form of T3 is not that great at helping with all the functions that the thyroid does.

The gut also has receptors for some neurotransmitters. If the gut is inflamed, then those neurotransmitters can't activate their receptors as well, and so you end up with GI symptoms. Some of them can be constipation, diarrhea, and weight gain.

I am often asked if I agree with or even know how to do a gut cleanse. I defer to nutrition experts on the how to. I do counsel to make sure that you are not just stripping away the protective mucous coating in the intestines. Also make sure you are replenishing your microbiome (gut bacteria) with the right balance.

The other component that will help you balance out your gut health and support your adrenal health and thyroid health is supplementation. Yes, we need vitamins, just like our kids. You need vitamins because even with eating a healthy diet, because the way our food sources are, they may not always have all the vitamins, minerals, and phytonutrients that they should have. Our diet is S.A.D. (Standard American Diet). And here is why. I remember growing up, my grandmother had a beautiful luscious garden that spanned the entire width of her backyard. She would have tomatoes, greens (turnips and collards), okra, bell peppers, cucumbers, pole beans, and sweet potatoes, just to name a few. I would notice that some years, she wouldn't plant as much or she would plant different items. I remember her talking about how you have to let the ground rest and replenish itself. This was so the soil would be able to give the right amount of nutrients to the foods and in turn to you.

Whew! I know I just gave you a lot of information to digest. Take a moment and take a few deep breaths. I mean breaths from your belly. The ones that make your shoulders relax. How do you feel? Do you feel validated? Yes, you did wake up in a body you don't recognize. Yes, people are getting on your last nerve. The good news is you are not alone, you are not crazy, and now you have a survival guide.

It has been a joy to share with you some tools that you will be able to use on your continued journey into the next phase of your womanhood.

Thank You Letter to My #BalancedBeauties

To all my balanced beauties. I want to thank you for entrusting your care to me over the years. It is because you have allowed me to be present at some of the most vulnerable times in your lives that I have been able to become such a laser-sharp integrative GYN and hormone specialist. And because of you, I have found another way to serve more ambitious woman who are struggling with depleting hormones get balanced, regain mental sharpness, and feel beautiful and vital again.

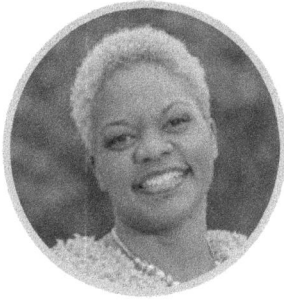

About the Author

Dr. LaKeischa Webb McMillan is an OB-GYN whose mission is to empower women for generations as they age to feel confident in knowing how balancing their hormones is essential to healthy living. Dr. LaKeischa graduated cum laude from Oakwood College, now Oakwood University, in Huntsville, Alabama, with a bachelor of science in biology, and earned her medical degree at Loma Linda University School of Medicine. As a mother, Dr. LaKeischa served as the PTA president at her kids' school and as a parent volunteer for the Silgo Adventurers Club in Takoma Park, Maryland. Her hobbies include hiking, swimming, and reading fiction. She lives in Silver Spring, Maryland, with her husband, Wendell II, and their two kids, Wendell III and Skylar Nicole.

Learn more at www.drlakeischamd.com

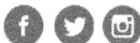